Testosterone

And miscellaneous stuff

Constantin Panow

To my parents, Kitcha and Pavel

"The Holy Supper is kept, indeed,

- In what so we share with another's need,

- Not that, which we give, but what we share,

- For the gift without the giver is bare."

*James Russel Lowell*

# Contents

A lot has been published in recent years on this topic.

Men of all countries, whether coming from sport endeavor, or just having aging problems, end-up being actively interested.

Thus, me as a professional in medicine, I receive every day publicity about a gimmick or some new regime, aiming at improving your T-level.

To make things clear from the beginning, let me tell you that there is no such thing as male hormones in blood!

In men between 20 and 45, testosterone level varies 4-fold, while the one of LH- 10 times between normal populations.

Ok, there is an overall tendency of plummeting with advancing age, but with personal comparisons in a controlled model this fact has never been challenged.

Despite huge literature in females, where a lot is known about sexual hormones, almost nothing is clearly depicted in papers about males.

So, for God's sake, would you tell me please, if female hormones are subjected to strong variations, and fluctuation being in itself warranty for function, why should it be so different in males?

Because, you would have heard already about the fact that every endocrine substance acts by attaching to a receptor, and in this respect there are two constants, the hormone itself, I agree, but also tissue sensitivity to it.

And this second one comes to exhaustion, if first variable is fixed and high all the time.

So, you would ask, where is the difference between men and women?

Well, this again is pretty simple!

While sexual gland release in blood has a half-life

of 4 hours for first, it is in vicinity of one whole day for second gender.

## Maximal plateau

Or, if you want to hear some less digestible stuff from my profession, to attain a steady-state, you need an average of 3.5 half-lives.

Thus, if you would like to conduct a study now in males, you should search for this fluctuation somewhere within 10-12 hours' time.

This is our physiologically predetermined ratio for a testosterone spurt to start its' down-slope.

## Physiology

Higher rates from that certain point on have a negative outcome on end-effect.

Thus, down-regulation of LH, which is secreted by hypophysis, and triggers testosterone secretion from interstitial, so-called Leydig's cells of testicles.

Testosterone is further metabolized and transformed by aromatase in fat-tissues, including the brain, in estradiol.

This one is a female hormone, with a half-life of 18-20 hours.

Three and a half times of this term, and we would have a natural cycle, if there wasn't interruption by daylight and its inner secretion, especially corticosteroids.

Adrenal interference is thus a very potent intermission, counteracting all other endocrinal glands.

## Illumination Deprivation

Thus, people who are living deep in caves, away from daylight, see their internal clock evolving with a recurrence of 3-4 days.

This is another issue obliging hibernating animals to gather more fat in their bodies, before retiring in some underground hollow for the snowy period, from where only warmth and strong sunlight of the new season wakes them up.

## Analogy

LH-testosterone-T-tissue-receptors can be analyzed as a chain very much similar to a spring coil.

A shorter spurt would produce a lower effect, while a longer one a higher end-result, till the end-point, which is probably in vicinity of 12-15 hours, from which onward you have again a lower outcome.

LH has a very short half-life, a few minutes only.

It has a negative downregulation with FSH, a similar secretion from adenohypophysis, but which is responsible for production of sperm by Sertoli's cells of testicles.

### Day-Night

Thus, you see our nyctohemera of 24 hours should be dedicated half to LH-testosterone and other 50% to FSH-spermatogenesis.

### Lyrics

If we try to envision this from the point of view of poetry, as scientific data are pretty scarce, we can say:

"Testosterone is the means of muscle, action, power, and day's vigilance, while female hormones are dedicated to the warmness of the night's bedroom…"

As you might know, spermatogenesis does not stop on external administration of testosterone, and such men remain to a high percentage fertile.

Owing to the fact that medication suppresses LH, but with a spurt of FSH.

## Motivation

Many men are dedicated to a life-long quest for muscle power, strength, trophicity and bulk.

Women are frequently attracted by such a physique, and besides it conveys the best an animal appearance in human outward.

This is such a strong trend, that many of our "weaker gender" companions start on a training program as well.

Their testosterone levels are not at all insignificant or inoperative, provided they would follow the "right" regime.

Not only their suprarenal glands secrete a small amount of it, but they convey also other androgens in their bodies.

For muscle growth main second pituitary secretion needed is growth hormone (GH).

This small peptide has a half-life of only minutes, like the two other ones released by the same adeno-hypophysis, LH and FSH.

Recent evidence points to the fact, that LH synthesis heavily depends on nutriments presented to cells.

Thus, sports communities conclude: -glucose!

And they implement it heavily in one's regime.

This has no adverse effects, the same as having several small meals during the day;

As long, as your body muscle out-weighs strongly body fat.

But, if organism lipids are prevalent, then aromatase transforms all androgens into estrogens, and you do not have the same muscle growth.

Don't forget in this respect, that starches were found to be main promoter of obesity epidemic in the States.

Sugars need insulin, a pancreas hormone, which

drives them into cells.

As long as it is heavily represented in blood stream, GH would be kept low.

If it goes down, as it would do on a fat diet, for instance, GH would have more chances to peak.

This is what trainers observe more and more world-wide.

GH is also linked to ghrelin, called also fasting hormone, as they go hand in hand.

### One between many?

A longer period of such withdrawal of food, does not mean that you can't get used to it.

One precedent is Hershel Walker, a professional American football player, who would eat only once per day;

And have an exceptional physique.

Ok, he is very skilled;

But he trains without any heavy weights at all;

Calisthenics only;

And he is vegetarian, consuming poultry once per month.

## Destruction

Another principles, which is probably exemplified here:

Is that, if you wish to burn fat, you consume lipids!

Does this mean, that if you eat proteins, you would catabolize muscle?

This is very much a probability...

As, we accelerate thus amino acids turn-over.

So, what?


## Practice

How should we nourish ourselves?

Training, we know already, should be anabolic one, brief, intense and compound!

Well, if you eat sugar, you engage your anatomy in a very short metabolic cycle.

At first a lot of glucose, insulin goes up, ghrelin and GH plummet;

Then, after only a short while, you have a rebound effect, as glucose, 4 kcal per gram, has been expended, and your body has to do with hypoglycemia.

And, you would say:

"You see, me too, I am fasting all the time!"

Yes, but you must consider that fat tissue has a very slow metabolism;

And if you want to burn lipids, you must give time to the machinery to start on lipolysis.

Besides, if we accustom it to be given sucrose, then it dissipates glucose accordingly.

## Different types of nutriments

Starches are very near to white sugar, having a glycemic index (GI) of 1, or almost.

Thus, consuming, bread, pasta, rice and potatoes is not far from first scenario.

French fries are the farthest from this, with a GI of 0.75.

This is because of all the oil they contain, which slows down stomach emptying.

There are potatoes out there, which are small and succulent, and if eaten with the pealing, (also with a good taste), have a GI of 0.5.

Also, if you consume them raw, this value falls even lower than this.

You see, how important New French Cuisine is, teaching us to cook little our vegetables!

## Philosophy

So, you see, as a friend of mine would put it:

"There is no such thing as a bad food, there are only evil people!"

Which my mother-in-law, Jeanne, would question, saying:

"There are only sufferers in this world!"

Bigger, and smaller?

But, this again, from a more neutral perspective, is very relative, and a matter of appreciation.

## Two types

But, apart from that, we have to do with two types of carbohydrates (CH):

Starch-CH and Fiber-CH.

Second ones are represented by vegetables and fresh salad.

So, if you are aiming at attaining proficiency of a highly qualified football player, accustom your body little by little to this second type of CH.

Horses perform very well, being fed only grass.

### Border ones

Green peas, green and snap beans and lentils belong to this group, though if you cook them long enough they would release a starch-like product in their broth.

So, we can use our organism to fasting little by little, emphasis being stressed on slow progression, reducing at first starches, then cutting them away completely from our diet.

### Intestinal failure

Animal studies report bilirubin gall-stones when adding 40% of fat to one's meals.

Depletion in biliary salts ensues with malabsorption syndrome.

This study in mice has been obtained with Starch-CH as second nutriment.

With Fiber-CH you would have more freedom increasing lipids, as first nutriment!

As, those ones are not promoting acceleration of bowel's peristalsis, as it was believed earlier, but a slowing down, as recent publications demonstrated!

Constipation being the result, and not diarrhea!

So, if we try to conclude this short overview, LH-testosterone secretion is promoted by proteins>sugars, while GH release- by fasting>lipid consume.

Both are counteracted by cortisol- the catabolic "stress" hormone!

This last one peaks in the morning hours, but rapidly drops down during the day.

It depends heavily on light intensity.

My second aim in this short booklet concerns athletes of the running community;

Whether long-distance or medium one. (Marathon practitioners).

Medical doctors, we see more and more cases of these sportsmen and –women, presenting with heavy atherosclerosis and even pseudo-gout.

How come?

As aerobics has been advocated for decades as a health improvement method!

### Traumatic lesions?

They suffer also frequently from so-called muscle tear.

You would say, this is obvious why!

But, my long practice, almost 40 years, teaches me otherwise.

This accident happens not when they are running full-pace, but often when exercising gently, or even walking!

### Ultrasound

As a radiologist, I have to analyze images, and what I saw led me to think that it's not muscle, which comes apart, but its envelope, or so-called fascia, or even tendons themselves.

For 10 years I was analyzing this issue, without finding the answer.

And then, one day it became obvious to me, that it had to do with nutrition.

Of course, after multiple discussions with patients about their habits and life-style!

Yes, apart from marathon runners, there is another community concerned, and guess what?

It is Mediterraneans!

Because they consume olive oil as only vegetal fat!

Who invented the theory that Greek population lives longer?

Many people in Switzerland outlast beyond.

But, don't misunderstand me, eating starches shortens one's endurance and vegetables, - lengthens it…

Besides, stress is very deleterious to our health!

But, enough for this preamble!

Let's start with the main points of our discussion.

Tendons and muscle sleeves (fasciae) are composed by extremely long cells, to adapt to anatomy.

This fact supposes a huge amount of membrane limiting the cytoplasm and its nucleus.

This one is constructed of phospholipids to a very high percentage (>90%).

Fats, in other words, and you need to provide to the body all nutritional elements needed, included omega 3, 5, 6, 7 etcetera, for its function and survival.

Especially, if those ones can't be synthesized by the human body.

If there is deficiency in some of those so-called essential fatty acids, cell membranes tear.

Another result, still poorly understood, with which we, as general practitioners, have to struggle very often;

Is prescription of medication, which lowers cholesterol in blood, and this despite the patient has normal values, or even, which is worse there are for instance side-effects like hepatitis.

### Labs again

HDL, LDL and VLDL are laboratory findings and can't imply body stores of circulating lipids.

What we know, is that HDL is responsible for taking away fat from periphery, while LDL bring it to cells.

### Negative

In other words, if you deprive by all means the body from some of its constituents, you impinge heavily on its metabolism.

### Storage

As essential fatty acids can be stored only for short periods of time, afterwards, they become triglycerides.

And main nutriment can't be transported any longer!

### Calculi again

Old publications already observed, that low fat

supply would end-up in more cholesterol gall-bladder stones.

And recent literature says, that the outcome of more lipids in meals is a lower body weight, and a leaner physique.

Adding essential fatty acids to one's meals would reverse even liver steatosis, pretends a recent article.

### Exceptions

In some areas, where fresh salad, vegetables and fruit are not readily available, supplements of essential fatty acids in recommended dosage doesn't change outcome of peripheral atherosclerosis, probably owing to high starch and meat consume.

### Conclusion

So, I would conclude, saying, that if you don't provide your anatomy with omega 3, 5, 6, 7, 9, and enough saturated and mono-unsaturated fat, you risk to end-up with over-training manifestations, burn-out, supra-renal exhaustion, and atherosclerosis.

This seems to me to be a rule to be followed, if you have already a lean physique, and are not suffering from metabolic syndrome, or in other words, pre-diabetes, of course!

Here I must remind you, that testosterone, and cortisol are formed from cholesterol.

And what about your brain, which is also more than 90% phospholipids?

While cholesterol can be synthesized only to a small percentage by the human body!

So, we depend largely to be provided from the outside.

Variety of fats proposed to the body should be also probably stressed.

*Website*

I hope, you enjoyed this short text.

If you have any comments, or questions, do not hesitate, write in my blog!

You can join me at:

www.thenopillshealthprospect.com